Rare Genetic Disorders

A Practical Guide to progeria and
Lesch-Nyhan syndrome.

Dr. Gerrard Andrews

Table of Contents

Introduction

Lesch-Nyhan syndrome and progeria are uncommon hereditary illnesses that afflict people all over the world. A hypoxanthine-guanine phosphoribosyltransferase (HGPRT) enzyme deficiency causes Lesch-Nyhan syndrome, which results in neurological and behavioral problems. Progeria is caused by a mutation in the LMNA gene, which results in premature aging.

The genetic cause of these disorders, their clinical presentations, and possible therapies have all been clarified by recent research. The diagnosis of rare genetic illnesses in children is increasingly being done through genomic testing, and the evidence supporting long-term adoption is mounting. Current research projects, such as gene therapy and small-molecule therapies, are intended to expedite the discovery of drugs for the treatment of various ailments. With organizations and activities uniting the rare illness community, increasing awareness, and fostering worldwide collaboration, collaborative efforts and global awareness in the field of rare genetic disorders have acquired substantial momentum.

For people and families impacted by these uncommon genetic illnesses, there are advocacy groups and supportive resources that offer tools, knowledge, and assistance in coping with the particular difficulties brought on by these illnesses. For people and families impacted by rare genetic disorders, quality of life and holistic care approaches—which include individualized care plans, access to resources and support networks, and a multidisciplinary care team—are crucial.

In conclusion, there is hope for better outcomes and therapies for those impacted by rare genetic disorders, thanks to the continued research and cooperative efforts in this area. Research on rare genetic disorders has a bright future thanks to developments in diagnosis, medication development, and discovery, as well as cooperative efforts and exciting new projects.

- **Definition of Rare Genetic Disorders**

A collection of unusual medical illnesses known as rare genetic disorders are caused by genetic abnormalities that impact one or more genes. These conditions fall into several groups, including X-linked, dominant, and recessive. Less than 200,000 Americans are afflicted with them, and they are typically less well-known or well-documented than more prevalent diseases, which makes them uncommon.

Important features of uncommon genetic illnesses include the following:

1. Causes: Mutations affecting one or more genes can result in rare genetic disorders, which can cause a variety of symptoms and health issues. These mutations may be complex (polygenic), chromosomal, or single-gene.

2. Types: There are various classifications for rare genetic illnesses, including dominant, recessive, and X-linked. Regardless of the existence of a healthy gene copy, dominant

illnesses arise when a mutation in a single gene is sufficient to produce the disorder. In recessive disorders, the disorder cannot appear unless both gene copies are mutated. When the mutation is found on the X chromosome, X-linked diseases result.

3. Inheritance: Depending on the nature of the condition, rare genetic disorders might be inherited by their progeny from their biological parents. Recessive disorders, on the other hand, are inherited from both parents, whereas dominant illnesses might be inherited from either parent.

4. Symptoms and Diagnosis: There is a wide spectrum of symptoms and health issues associated with rare genetic illnesses, which can present in different ways. A patient's medical history, physical examination, and genetic testing to determine whether a mutation is present are usually used in the diagnosis process.

5. Treatment and Management: Depending on the particular condition and its symptoms,

there are several approaches to treating and managing uncommon genetic disorders. Certain rare genetic disorders may not have a cure, but there are a number of techniques that can assist patients and their families in managing their symptoms, enhancing their quality of life, and getting supportive care.

6. Research and Future Directions: Research on uncommon genetic illnesses attempts to enhance diagnosis and therapy by enhancing our knowledge of their causes and effects. Researching these conditions can shed light on innovative biological processes and aid in the creation of fresh remedies for prevalent illnesses in people.

- **Significance of Studying Progeria and Lesch-Nyhan Syndrome**

Researching uncommon genetic conditions like Lesch-Nyhan syndrome and progeria is crucial because of their distinct traits, effects on the afflicted people, and insights they offer into more general aspects of genetic and molecular biology.

Hutchinson-Gilford Progeria Syndrome, or progeria

Hutchinson-Gilford Progeria syndrome (HGPS), also known as progeria, is an exceedingly rare and fatal genetic illness that causes children to age rapidly. Progerin is an aberrant protein that is produced as a result of a spontaneous autosomal dominant mutation in the LMNA gene. There are an estimated 400 children living with HGPS worldwide, and the illness is prevalent in about 1 in 20 million people. The gene alteration is hardly ever inherited, and the mutation nearly invariably happens by accident.

Lesch-Nyhan Syndrome

Males are mostly affected by Lesch-Nyhan syndrome (LNS), a rare X-linked recessive genetic condition. Hypoxanthine-guanine phosphoribosyltransferase (HGPRT) is an enzyme that is either significantly reduced or absent due to mutati. LNS affects roughly 1 in

380,000 people, and it nearly always affects boys in their early years.

Importance of Researching These Conditions

1. Insights into Genetic Mechanisms: Studies on Lesch-Nyhan Syndrome and Progeria offer important new perspectives on the molecular and genetic processes underlying these diseases. Gaining insight into certain gene mutations and their consequences advances our understanding of genetic disorders and possible treatment avenues.

2. Development of Therapies: Researchers can find possible treatments for Lesch-Nyhan syndrome and progeria by examining these uncommon genetic disorders. These treatments may also have effects on other conditions that are related to these two rare genetic disorders. For example, the identification of progerin in progeria has provided insight into the aging process and possible therapies for ailments associated with aging.

3. Clinical Management and Support: Improving patient treatment, creating supportive interventions, and raising the standard of living for impacted persons and their families all depend on an understanding of the clinical signs and disease progression of Progeria and Lesch-Nyhan Syndrome.

In summary, research on uncommon genetic diseases like Lesch-Nyhan syndrome and progeria not only advances our knowledge of and ability to treat these particular ailments, but it also has wider ramifications for genetic research, the development of new treatments, and clinical care. These illnesses are significant subjects for scientific inquiry and medical advancement due to their distinct genetic and clinical traits.

Chapter One

Hutchinson-Gilford Progeria Syndrome

Hutchinson-Gilford Children with Progeria Syndrome (HGPS) exhibit accelerated aging as a result of this rare genetic condition. Its incidence is roughly one per eight million live births, and its cause is a mutation in the LMNA gene. At birth, children with HGPS usually have normal appearances, but with time, they have slower growth, hair loss, skin that looks aged, and unique facial traits, including large eyes and a small chin. Both motor skills and intellectual development are unaffected by the condition. Every case of progeria is deadly, typically as a result of heart attacks or strokes. Since it is an autosomal dominant disorder, the illness can be brought on by just one mutant copy of the gene in each cell. While there isn't a known treatment for HGPS, managing the condition focuses on symptom relief and providing support to the impacted kids and their families.

1.1 Overview and History

An uncommon genetic condition called Hutchinson-Gilford Progeria Syndrome (HGPS) is characterized by children who age rapidly. Hutchinson-Gilford progeria syndrome was subsequently termed after it was initially identified by Jonathan Hutchinson in 1886 and independently by Hastings Gilford in 1897. The disorder is brought on by a mutation in the LMNA gene, which results in the production of the Lamin A protein and causes the cell nucleus to become structurally unstable, accelerating the aging process. At birth, children with HGPS usually have normal appearances, but as they get older, they often exhibit slower growth, hair loss, skin that seems older, and unique facial traits. The illness is always fatal, usually as a result of heart attacks or strokes. It is an autosomal dominant disorder, meaning that one copy of the defective gene in each cell is sufficient to cause the syndrome, and it affects about 1 in 8 million live births. Although HGPS has no known cure, treatment aims to support afflicted children and their families while reducing symptoms.

1.2 Genetic Basis and Inheritance

Hutchinson-Gilford An aberrant protein termed progerin is produced as a result of a de novo point mutation in the LMNA gene, which causes Progeria Syndrome (HGPS), a rare genetic condition. Children affected by this mutation experience quick and severe aging. Since HGPS is regarded as an autosomal dominant disorder, the disorder can be caused by a single mutant copy of the gene in each cell.

The rare nature of HGPS inheritance makes it distinct from other inheritance patterns. Children that are affected never survive long enough to have children of their own, and it is typically caused by a new (sporadic) mutation that occurs during the early division of the cells. Even though this is not the usual pattern, the extremely small number of documented cases of afflicted siblings raises the possibility of an autosomal recessive inheritance.

Hutchinson-Gilford progeria syndrome was the term given to the illness when it was initially identified by Jonathan Hutchinson in 1886 and independently by Hastings Gilford in 1897. It is characterized by the dramatic, rapid aging process that starts in childhood. Affected children usually look normal at birth and in the early stages of infancy, but as time goes on, they grow slower, lose hair, and acquire distinctive facial features that are indicative of an aged appearance.

To summarize, the main cause of Hutchinson-Gilford Progeria Syndrome is a de novo point mutation in the LMNA gene, which results in the aberrant protein progerin being produced. Even though it is usually classified as an autosomal dominant disorder, affected children hardly ever survive long enough to become parents. It is also practically never handed on from parent to child.

1.3 Clinical Features and Symptoms

Hutchinson-Gilford An uncommon genetic condition known as progeria syndrome (HGPS) affects about 1 in 8 million live births. A de novo point mutation in the LMNA gene is the cause, and it results in the erroneous protein known as progerin. The disorder is typified by the affected children aging quickly, usually starting in early childhood. At birth, children with HGPS typically have normal appearances, but as they get older, they often exhibit slower growth, hair loss, skin that seems older, and unique facial traits, including large eyes and a small chin.

In addition, they have weakening bones, a high-pitched voice, and cardiovascular issues, which account for the majority of their deaths. Intellectual development and motor skills remain unaffected, despite the physical symptoms. Affected children hardly ever survive long enough to become parents themselves, and the ailment is nearly never handed down from parent to child. Although HGPS has no known cure, treatment aims to support afflicted children and their families while reducing symptoms. The quality of life and survival rate of HGPS can be improved by an interdisciplinary team's early diagnosis and care.

1.4 Diagnosis and Genetic Testing

Hutchinson-Gilford Progeria syndrome (HGPS) diagnosis is made through a combination of genetic testing and clinical assessment. Suspicion of HGPS might arise from its clinical symptoms, which include delayed growth, hair loss, aged-looking skin, and distinctive facial features. However, in order to confirm the diagnosis, genetic testing is required. A de novo point mutation in the LMNA gene, which results in the atypical protein progerin's synthesis, is the genetic basis of HGPS.

Comprehensive genomic testing is required for HGPS genetic testing in order to pinpoint the precise LMNA gene mutation. For children suspected of having HGPS, the Progeria Research Foundation offers a DNA-based diagnostic test in collaboration with a CLIA-approved diagnostics lab. With the use of this test, children with HGPS can be definitively diagnosed because it pinpoints the precise LMNA gene mutation.

It is significant to remember that classical HGPS is typically caused by a novel, rare mutation that occurs during the early stages of cell division and is hardly ever passed down from parent to child. Consequently, healthy parents typically won't give it to their kids. Seldom do impacted children survive long enough to become parents.

To sum up, the process of diagnosing HGPS entails assessing the syndrome's distinctive characteristics clinically. Subsequently, genetic testing is employed to pinpoint the precise mutation in the LMNA gene, thereby validating the diagnosis.

1.5 Current Treatment Options

Hutchinson-Gilford Children with Progeria Syndrome (HGPS) exhibit accelerated aging as a result of this rare genetic condition. As of right now, there is no known cure for HGPS; instead, treatment plans concentrate on symptom relief and providing support to impacted children and their families. The following are some HGPS therapy options:

1. Standard of care: growth hormone therapy, dietary assistance, and management of consequences like cardiac problems and joint stiffness are among the best forms of care provided to patients with HGPS in order to treat the signs and symptoms.

2. Zokinvy: A medicine called lonafarnib has been licensed by the FDA to be used as the initial treatment for children with HGPS who are one year of age or older. It has been demonstrated that lonafarnib, a particular inhibitor of farnesyltransferase (FTI), inhibits the production of aberrant progerin, a protein that speeds up the aging process in HGPS. Zokinvy comes in hard capsule form and is taken twice daily.

3. Early intervention: Children with HGPS have a higher chance of survival and a better quality of life when early intervention is provided by a multidisciplinary team. This could involve growth hormone treatment, routine examinations, and problem-solving techniques.

4. Support and counseling: Organizations like the Progeria Research Foundation, which links families with impacted children, raises money for research, and speaks out for the needs of the children and their families, frequently offer support and counseling to families affected by HGPS.

To summarize, the standard of care, Zokinvy, early intervention, and support and counseling for afflicted children and their families are available as therapy options for Hutchinson-Gilford Progeria Syndrome. Although there isn't a cure for HGPS, these therapies can help kids with the condition live better and manage their symptoms.

1.6 Ongoing Research and Future Therapeutic Avenues

Future therapy approaches for Hutchinson-Gilford Progeria Syndrome (HGPS) and ongoing research are centered on creating medications to control the condition's symptoms and maybe halt the aging process in afflicted youngsters. The following are a few of the present study avenues and possible treatment strategies:

1. Zokinvy: The first FDA-approved treatment for children with HGPS one year of age and older is Zokinvy, a medicine that contains lonafarnib. A particular farnesyltransferase (FTI) inhibitor called lonsafarnib stops aberrant progerin from forming, which is a protein that accelerates aging in HGPS.

2. Isoprenylcysteine Carboxylmethyltransferase-Based Therapy: This promising therapeutic strategy attempts to address the cellular and molecular alterations brought on by progerin buildup, including aberrant DDR and nuclear abnormalities.

3. Gene Therapy: To address the mutation in the LMNA gene that causes HGPS, researchers are looking at the possibilities of utilizing gene therapy. This strategy might result in a treatment for the illness.

4. Epigenetic Modulation: It has been determined that epigenetic changes, such as DNA methylation and histone alterations, may be useful treatment targets for HGPS. In children who are affected, these alterations may help slow down the aging process by changing the expression of certain genes.

5. Nucleoside Replacement Therapy: This method attempts to fix the damaged nucleosides in HGPS-affected children's cells, which may help with some of the syndrome's symptoms.

Hutchinson-Gilford Progeria syndrome is being studied further, and potential treatment options include nucleoside replacement therapy, gene therapy, isoprenylcysteine carboxylmethyltransferase-based therapy, Zokinvy, and epigenetic regulation. These prospective therapies seek to control the symptoms and maybe delay the aging process in impacted youngsters, enhancing their chances of survival and quality of life.

Chapter Two

Lesch-Nyhan Syndrome

Lesch-Nyhan syndrome is an uncommon hereditary illness that primarily impacts men. Neurological and behavioral problems result from a deficit in the enzyme hypoxanthine-guanine phosphoribosyltransferase (HGPRT). Severe gout, poor muscle control, mild developmental deficits, and self-injury—the most prevalent and characteristic behavioral component of the condition—are among the symptoms of Lesch-Nyhan syndrome.

Genetic testing can identify whether a person has acquired the mutation that causes Lesch-Nyhan syndrome, which is inherited as an X-linked recessive genetic disorder. Lesch-Nyhan syndrome affects about 1 in 380,000 people and is present in all populations at a similar frequency.

Lesch-Nyhan syndrome's neurological symptoms have no established course of treatment; instead, care is mostly symptomatic. Allopurinol, which regulates high uric acid levels, can be used to treat gout. Lithotripsy, which uses shock waves or laser beams to break up kidney stones, can be used to treat kidney stones. The medications haloperidol, diazepam, phenobarbital, and carbidopa/levodopa may help with some of the neurological symptoms.

In conclusion, neurological and behavioral problems are the result of Lesch-Nyhan syndrome, a rare hereditary illness that almost exclusively affects boys. Supportive care and symptomatic treatment can help control symptoms and enhance the quality of life for those who are affected, even though there is no conventional treatment for the neurological symptoms of the disorder.

2.1 Introduction and Background

Males are typically affected by Lesch-Nyhan syndrome (LNS), a rare genetic condition that is inherited as an X-linked recessive genetic disorder. Hypoxanthine-guanine phosphoribosyltransferase (HPRT) deficiency is the disorder's etiology, as it causes an excess of uric acid to be produced in all bodily fluids. Acute gouty arthritis, reduced renal function, and self-mutilating habits like biting one's lips, fingers, or skull are all signs of liposuction syndrome (LNS). Self-mutilation is the most notable aspect of LNS, and it has been seen in about 85% of patients. Most frequently, these behaviors start when a child is two or three years old.

On the other hand, some patients are intelligent enough. The neurological symptoms of LNS do not have a conventional course of treatment, although there are strategies to help control the symptoms and lower their consequences. Allopurinol, which regulates high uric acid levels, can be used to treat gout. Lithotripsy, which uses shock waves or laser beams to break up kidney stones, can be used to treat kidney stones.

2.2 Genetic Basis and X-Linked Recessive Inheritance

Males are typically affected by Lesch-Nyhan syndrome (LNS), a rare genetic ailment that is inherited as an X-linked recessive condition. The hypoxanthine-guanine phosphoribosyltransferase (HPRT) enzyme deficiency that causes the condition causes an excess of uric acid to be produced in all bodily fluids. Males with only one X chromosome are more likely to be affected by the condition due to the X-linked recessive inheritance pattern, which indicates that the affected gene is situated on the X chromosome.

Mutations in the HPRT1 gene, which is situated at the q26–27 location on the long arm of the X chromosome, are linked to the genetic basis of LNS. More than 600 mutations have been found, and each one causes clinical manifestations that range in severity. Males are nearly entirely affected by the condition, with female carriers occurring in the majority of cases. But if the normal X chromosome has a mutation and the faulty X chromosome manifests phenotypically, females may also get the illness.

The estimated prevalence of LNS as stated earlier is 1 in 380,000 people. Males with the syndrome are affected from birth, and symptoms include significant developmental impairments, poor muscle control, and severe gout. Self-mutilating behaviors, which can include head banging and biting of the lips and fingers, are the most noticeable aspect of LNS. LNS is treated symptomatically, with lithotripsy used to cure kidney stones and allopurinol used to decrease high uric acid levels in the gout patient. The neurological symptoms of LNS do not have a conventional course of treatment, yet certain drugs may be able to ease particular symptoms.

2.3   Clinical   Manifestations   and Behavioral Symptoms

Lesch-Nyhan syndrome (LNS) is an uncommon hereditary condition marked by excess uric acid production as well as anomalies in the nervous system and behavior. The syndrome is inherited as an X-linked recessive disorder that mainly affects men. The overproduction of uric acid resulting from a lack of the enzyme hypoxanthine-guanine phosphoribosyltransferase (HPRT) causes symptoms such as acute gouty arthritis, poor kidney function, and self-mutilating behaviors. Lip and finger biting as well as head bashing are examples of self-injury, which is the most prevalent and recognizable behavioral manifestation of LNS. Severe developmental difficulties, neurological dysfunction, and involuntary muscular movements are further signs. The prognosis for LNS is typically poor, and the neurological symptoms are frequently severe. LNS affects roughly 1 in 380,000 people, and in males, the disorder is present from birth. A defining characteristic of LNS is self-injury, and those who experience it typically need assistance with everyday tasks and mobility. Almost solely in males is the disease diagnosed, since female bearers of the genetic mutation usually do not exhibit any symptoms. The X chromosome contains the genetic mutation that causes LNS. Those who are affected have a severe lack or shortage of the HPRT enzyme, which results in a variety of behavioral and clinical symptoms.

The most prevalent and defining behavioral characteristic of LNS is self-mutilation, which is one of its behavioral symptoms. This self-harming activity is typified by head banging, biting of the lips and fingers, and other self-harming behaviors. People with LNS may also engage in involuntary muscle movements, such as dystonia, choreoathetosis, and ballismus, in addition to self-mutilation. Movement and the ability to carry out daily tasks might be severely hampered by certain movement disorders. The prognosis for those with LNS is typically dismal, and the neurological symptoms are frequently severe. Kidney stones, severe gouty arthritis, and reduced kidney function can all be signs of LNS's overproduction of uric acid.

The substantial effects of LNS on afflicted individuals and their families are largely due to the confluence of uric acid overproduction, neurological abnormalities, and behavioral abnormalities.

In conclusion, Lesch-Nyhan syndrome is an uncommon hereditary disease marked by an excess of uric acid production along with a variety of clinical symptoms, such as neurological and behavioral problems. The syndrome is inherited as an X-linked recessive disorder that mainly affects men. The primary behavioral indicator of lip and finger biting, head banging, and other self-harming behaviors is known as self-mutilation (LNS). The condition has a substantial impact on affected individuals and their families because it is linked to severe developmental delays, involuntary muscular spasms, and poor renal function.

2.4 Diagnostic Approaches and Genetic Testing

Rare genetic disorder Lesch-Nyhan syndrome (LNS) is inherited as an X-linked recessive illness and is virtually exclusively diagnosed in males. Clinical signs, such as problems in the nervous system and behavior, together with an excess of uric acid, are used to diagnose LNS. Specific blood tests, such as measuring uric acid levels and the HPRT enzyme's activity, can confirm the diagnosis of LNS. By detecting changes in the HPRT1 gene, genetic testing can also be utilized to validate the diagnosis of LNS. Amniocentesis or chorionic villus samples can be used for prenatal diagnosis in order to identify if the developing fetus has the HPRT1 mutation. Because of the wide range of clinical symptoms and comorbidity with other neurological and behavioral illnesses, the diagnosis of LNS is frequently difficult. For the diagnosis and treatment of LNS, a multidisciplinary approach comprising neurologists, geneticists, and behavioral specialists is advised.

In conclusion, Lesch-Nyhan syndrome is diagnosed based on clinical signs such as excess uric acid production and abnormalities of the nervous system and behavior. The diagnosis of LNS can be verified by specialized blood tests, such as those that detect uric acid levels and the activity of the HPRT enzyme. HPRT1 gene mutations can also be found by genetic testing. Amniocentesis or chorionic villus samples can be used to diagnose pregnancies. For the diagnosis and treatment of LNS, a multidisciplinary approach is advised due to the diversity of clinical presentations and the overlap with other neurological and behavioral disorders.

2.5 Management and Supportive Care

Lesch-Nyhan syndrome (LNS) is a rare genetic illness that primarily affects men. It is characterized by anomalies in the nervous system and behavior, as well as an excess production of uric acid. LNS has no known cure; symptoms are managed with supportive care. A multidisciplinary team consisting of neurologists, geneticists, and behavioral specialists manages LNS. The goal of LNS treatment is to control symptoms and minimize side effects. Allopurinol, which regulates high uric acid levels, can be used to treat gout. Lithotripsy, which uses shock waves or laser beams to break up kidney stones, can be used to treat kidney stones. The neurological symptoms of LNS do not have a conventional course of treatment; however, certain drugs may be able to lessen certain symptoms. To treat dystonia, choreoathetosis, and ballismus, for instance, medications such as haloperidol, diazepam, phenobarbital, and carbidopa/levodopa may be utilized. Protective equipment, behavioral therapy, and physical constraints can all be used to manage behavioral symptoms like self-harm. Individuals with LNS require supportive treatment, and families may find that attending counseling sessions and support groups is beneficial.

In conclusion, there is no known cure for Lesch-Nyhan syndrome, and treatment options are limited to symptomatic and supportive measures. The goals of treatment are to control the symptoms and minimize side effects. Allopurinol is a treatment for gout, while lithotripsy is a treatment for kidney stones. The neurological symptoms of LNS do not have a conventional course of treatment; however, certain drugs may be able to lessen certain symptoms. Protective equipment, behavioral therapy, and physical constraints can all be used to manage behavioral symptoms like self-harm. Individuals with LNS require supportive treatment, and families may find that attending counseling sessions and support groups is beneficial.

2.6 Research Advances and Potential Therapies

The goal of research on Lesch-Nyhan Syndrome (LNS) has been to comprehend the disorder's genetic and metabolic underpinnings and investigate possible treatment strategies. Mutations in the HPRT1 gene result in a deficit of the enzyme hypoxanthine-guanine phosphoribosyltransferase (HPRT), which causes LNS. There are more than 600 known mutations that cause different degrees of clinical severity.

Current studies have looked into the genotypic and phenotypic range of LNS, as well as how compensatory mechanisms and residual enzymes affect the disease's clinical severity. In an effort to comprehend the connection between genetic variants and the clinical manifestation of the condition, research has also looked into possible genotype-phenotype correlations in LNS.

Regarding possible treatments, studies have looked at fresh perspectives on LNS, such as looking into presynaptic dopaminergic deficiencies and using medication to address behavioral problems linked to the syndrome. Certain drugs have been used to treat behavioral symptoms in certain patients, including carbamazepine, baclofen, gabapentin, and depakote (sodium valproate). Additionally, studies have shown how crucial genetic counseling is for parents of children with LNS.

All things considered, LNS research has advanced our knowledge of the underlying genetic and metabolic processes of the illness and aided in the creation of viable treatment plans. However, additional study is required to improve our understanding of the illness and investigate cutting-edge therapy options.

Chapter Three

A Comparative Analysis

Progeria and Lesch-Nyhan syndrome (LNS) are two uncommon hereditary diseases with different features. A lack of the enzyme HPRT1 results in an X-linked recessive condition called LNS, which manifests as uncontrollably self-harming, intellectual impairment, and mobility issues. Males are the most affected, and there are no basic therapeutic options. Conversely, progeria, sometimes called Hutchinson-Gilford progeria syndrome, is an uncommon genetic disorder that causes children to age quickly. Symptoms include stunted growth, hair and body fat loss, wrinkles, and stiff joints.

Progeria is linked to a mutation in the LMNA gene, whereas LNS is caused by mutations in the HPRT1 gene. Using CRISPR-mediated base and prime editing, recent research has investigated therapeutic gene correction for LNS, providing possible treatment routes for this debilitating hereditary disease. Progeria, on the other hand, has no known cure; therefore, treatment for the illness concentrates on symptom relief and enhancing quality of life.

In conclusion, progeria and LNS are uncommon genetic illnesses with different etiologies and clinical presentations. While developments in gene editing hold out hope for the treatment of leukemia, supportive care is still the mainstay of progeria management.

3.1 Variations in Genetic Etiology

Lesch-Nyhan syndrome and progeria are two uncommon genetic diseases with different genetic etiologies. Mutations in the HPRT1 gene result in a deficit of the enzyme HPRT1, which causes an abnormal build-up of uric acid in the blood, which is the cause of Lesch-Nyhan syndrome (LNS). However, a mutation in the LMNA gene, which codes for the lamin A protein, is linked to progeria and results in the formation of progerin, a poisonous protein. Children who are on progesterone experience accelerated aging, which results in characteristics like stunted growth, hair and body fat loss, wrinkles that look older, and stiff joints.

Recent studies have investigated CRISPR-mediated base and prime editing as a therapeutic gene correction method for LNS, providing a possible treatment pathway for this debilitating hereditary disease. Progeria, on the other hand, has no known cure; therefore, treatment for the illness concentrates on symptom relief and enhancing quality of life.

In conclusion, progeria and LNS have different genetic etiologies, even though they are both uncommon genetic illnesses. While developments in gene editing hold out hope for the treatment of leukemia, supportive care is still the mainstay of progeria management.

3.2 Variability in Clinical Presentations

Lesch-Nyhan syndrome and progeria are two uncommon genetic diseases with different clinical manifestations. Progeria, sometimes referred to as Hutchinson-Gilford progeria syndrome, is a condition in which children age quickly, resulting in characteristics including stunted growth, hair and body fat loss, wrinkles that look older, and stiff joints. The usual life expectancy is approximately 15 years, and the condition is always fatal. On the other hand, excessive uric acid production, compulsive self-injury, and neurological and behavioral abnormalities are the hallmarks of Lesch-Nyhan syndrome (LNS). It typically manifests in the first year of life and mainly affects male children.

A genetic mutation in the LMNA gene, which codes for the lamin A protein, is the primary cause of the clinical signs of progeria, which include fast aging and unique physical characteristics. On the other hand, a lack of the enzyme HPRT1 is associated with the symptoms of Lesch-Nyhan syndrome, which results in an excess of uric acid and neurological abnormalities.

Lesch-Nyhan syndrome is marked by neurological and behavioral problems, uncontrollably self-injurious conduct, and accelerated aging. In summary, progeria and

Lesch-Nyhan syndrome have different clinical presentations.

3.3 Distinctive Challenges and Care Considerations

Progeria and Lesch-Nyhan syndrome have different clinical presentations and etiologies, which make them unique conditions with special treatment requirements. Hutchinson-Gilford progeria syndrome (HGPS), another name for progeria, is an uncommon genetic disorder that causes children to age rapidly. Symptoms include stunted growth, hair and body fat loss, wrinkles that look older, and stiff joints. The typical life expectancy of the illness is approximately 15 years, and it is invariably deadly. Progeria has no known treatment, and its cause is a mutation in the LMNA gene.

Conversely, Lesch-Nyhan syndrome (LNS) is an incredibly rare metabolic illness that mainly affects boys. It causes significant anomalies in the nervous system and behavior, including compulsive self-harm, intellectual incapacity, and difficulties with locomotion. Lesch-Nyhan syndrome patients have a dismal prognosis; most of them rarely survive longer than 20 years as a result of illness complications. A mutation in the HPRT1 gene results in an excess of uric acid synthesis, which causes LNS.

The following are some of the unique difficulties and care factors for these conditions:

Since heart attacks and strokes caused by atherosclerosis account for the majority of progeria-related deaths in children, supportive care is necessary to manage symptoms, including cardiovascular complications.
Lesch-Nyhan syndrome requires continuous assistance, symptom management, and individualized treatment strategies to address the overproduction of uric acid, neurological abnormalities, and behavioral abnormalities.

In summary, the unique clinical symptoms and genetic etiologies of progeria and Lesch-Nyhan syndrome present specific challenges and care considerations that necessitate specialist assistance and management in order to enhance the quality of life for those who are affected.

Chapter Four

Living with Rare Genetic Disorders

Because uncommon genetic disorders like Lesch-Nyhan syndrome and progeria have different clinical presentations and genetic etiologies, living with them comes with unique problems. Progeria, sometimes referred to as Hutchinson-Gilford progeria syndrome, is a condition in which children age quickly, resulting in characteristics including stunted growth, hair and body fat loss, wrinkles that look older, and stiff joints.

The typical life expectancy of the illness is approximately 15 years, and it is invariably deadly. Conversely, Lesch-Nyhan syndrome (LNS) is an incredibly rare metabolic illness that mainly affects boys. It causes significant anomalies in the nervous system and behavior, including compulsive self-harm, intellectual incapacity, and difficulties with locomotion. Lesch-Nyhan syndrome patients have a dismal prognosis; most of them rarely survive longer than 20 years as a result of illness complications.

Managing the accompanying symptoms, addressing the impact on quality of life, and offering continuing support and care are among the difficulties of having these conditions. This may entail treating cardiovascular issues as well as the psychological and social effects of progeria on individuals. Managing the overproduction of uric acid, treating the neurological and behavioral problems, and offering support to the patient and their family are all important aspects of care for people with Lesch-Nyhan syndrome.

Access to specialist medical care, support services, and resources is crucial for individuals and their families facing rare genetic disorders in order to effectively manage the particular problems that come with them. While research on prospective medicines and treatments for rare genetic disorders is still ongoing, the present emphasis is on offering complete care and support to improve the quality of life for those who are affected.

In conclusion, managing the particular difficulties brought on by living with uncommon genetic diseases like progeria and Lesch-Nyhan syndrome calls for specialist treatment, continuous support, and access to resources. Even though the prognosis for these conditions is sometimes dismal, attempts are being made to enhance the outcomes and quality of life for those who suffer from uncommon genetic disorders.

4.1 Patient and Family Perspectives

For patients and their families, living with uncommon genetic illnesses like Lesch-Nyhan syndrome and progeria can bring particular problems. These diseases can have a major negative influence on an affected person's quality of life due to their unique clinical presentations and genetic etiologies.

In rare genetic illnesses, patient and family views include:

1. Knowing the illness: Families must be aware of the illness, its signs, and possible effects on their child's life. This might assist them in giving the right kind and amount of support.

2. Managing symptoms: Families need to collaborate closely with their child's medical professionals to address the symptoms of these disorders, which include uncontrollably damaging oneself, growth failure, loss of hair and body fat, skin that appears aged, stiff joints, abnormalities in the nervous system, and abnormal behavior.

3. Navigating the healthcare system: Parents of children with rare genetic disorders frequently have to go through convoluted systems to get their children the specialized care they require and to coordinate their care with that of several healthcare specialists.

4. Emotional support: Following a diagnosis, families may experience a sense of overwhelm

and turn to support groups, counseling, or other services for emotional support.

5. Advocacy and awareness: Families can help advance the knowledge and treatment of these illnesses by working with healthcare professionals and researchers, taking part in research efforts, and advocating for greater resources and awareness for the specific disorder that affects their child.

6. Creating individualized care plans: Medical professionals should collaborate with families to create individualized care plans that address the particular difficulties brought on by progeria and Lesch-Nyhan syndrome and adapt to the child's evolving needs.

7. Access to resources: educational materials, financial aid, and support services are just a few of the tools that families should have at their disposal to help them deal with the particular difficulties brought on by these conditions.

In conclusion, progeria and Lesch-Nyhan syndrome are examples of rare genetic conditions that can be difficult for patients and their families to live with. However, families can enhance the quality of life for their loved ones and more effectively manage the condition by learning about it, managing symptoms, navigating the healthcare system, seeking emotional support, advocating for awareness, creating personalized care plans, and utilizing resources.

4.2 Supportive Resources and Advocacy Organizations

For people and families impacted by uncommon genetic illnesses like progeria and Lesch-Nyhan syndrome, there are numerous advocacy groups and supporting resources accessible. These groups offer resources, information, and support to help people with these conditions and their families deal with the particular difficulties they face.

One such group is the International Lesch-Nyhan Disease Association, a self-help, non-profit group whose mission is to support and educate families whose children have Lesch-Nyhan syndrome. The group advocates on behalf of patients and raises awareness of the illness among medical professionals. Through its database, directory, article reprints, and brochures, it also provides a range of informational and support materials and facilitates the sharing of resources, information, and support among impacted families.

The Cleveland Clinic is an additional resource that offers support and information to people with Lesch-Nyhan syndrome and their families. In addition to providing continuous support and symptom alleviation, the clinic creates individualized care plans to match the evolving requirements of affected patients.

The Progeria Research Foundation is a non-profit organization that works to develop a cure and therapies for progeria that benefit affected individuals and their families. For impacted people and their families, the foundation offers resources and support, such as financial aid, educational materials, and access to clinical trials.

In summary, people and families impacted by uncommon genetic illnesses like progeria and Lesch-Nyhan syndrome have access to a number of advocacy groups and supporting resources. These groups offer resources, information, and support to help people with these conditions and their families deal with the particular difficulties they face.

4.3 Quality of Life and Holistic Care Approaches

For people and families impacted by uncommon genetic diseases, including progeria and Lesch-Nyhan syndrome, quality of life and holistic treatment techniques are crucial. Individuals with these conditions may experience substantial reductions in quality of life; nevertheless, a comprehensive approach to therapy can assist in symptom management and enhance general health.

Early diagnosis and treatment can enhance the quality of life for people with Lesch-Nyhan syndrome, and medical professionals can provide continuing support and symptom relief. Support services can assist families in navigating the healthcare system and obtaining resources, while a specific care plan can aid in managing neurological and behavioral abnormalities.

Supportive treatment can help progeria patients manage symptoms, including cardiovascular problems, and social and emotional support can help them deal with how the disease affects their quality of life. Numerous progeria symptoms have improved with therapy alternatives, including the medication lonafarnib, and current studies are looking into possible gene therapies and small-molecule treatments.

For uncommon genetic illnesses, holistic care methods take into account social, emotional, and physical requirements. This may entail treating the psychological effects of the illness on afflicted people and their families, as well as facilitating access to resources, support services, and specialist medical care. A multidisciplinary care team can assist in symptom management, offer afflicted people emotional support, and enhance their general quality of life.

In conclusion, quality of life and comprehensive methods of care are critical for people with uncommon genetic illnesses like Lesch-Nyhan syndrome and progeria, as well as their families. Having a multidisciplinary care team, a tailored care plan, and access to resources and services can help control symptoms, attend to social and emotional needs, and enhance general wellbeing.

Chapter Five

Future Directions and Research Prospects

Prospects for future study and directions in uncommon genetic illnesses like Lesch-Nyhan syndrome and progeria include the following:

1. Gene therapy: Although this therapy is still in development and is not yet widely utilized, researchers are investigating the possibility of using gene therapy to correct harmful mutations in progeria. In the future, gene therapy might prove to be a beneficial therapeutic alternative.

2. Small molecule treatments: Research on progeria small molecule therapeutics is still ongoing. These treatments may help control symptoms and enhance the lives of those who are affected.

3. Clinical studies: In an effort to investigate possible cures and treatments for this uncommon genetic illness, the Progeria

Research Foundation is developing and funding clinical trials for people with progeria.

4. Advocacy and awareness: Groups like the Progeria Research Foundation and the International Lesch-Nyhan Disease Association are trying to spread the word about these uncommon genetic disorders and push for more funding and assistance for the people who are impacted by them and their families.

5. Personalized care plans: In order to address the particular difficulties posed by progeria and Lesch-Nyhan syndrome, healthcare professionals are creating customized care plans that offer continuing support and symptom relief.

In conclusion, research prospects and future directions in rare genetic disorders like Lesch-Nyhan syndrome and progeria include investigating gene therapy, small-molecule treatments, clinical trials, advocacy, and raising awareness. Personalized care plans are also being developed to help affected individuals manage their symptoms and live better lives.

5.1 Emerging Therapeutic Strategies

Clinical data and recent studies have shown new treatment approaches for uncommon genetic illnesses like Lesch-Nyhan syndrome and progeria. Various approaches offer hope for better management and therapy by addressing the distinct clinical presentations and genetic foundations of various disorders. The following are some new treatment approaches and areas of potential future research for these uncommon genetic illnesses:

Progeria:

1. Gene Therapy: Although this method is still in development and has not yet gained widespread use, research is looking at the possibility of directly repairing harmful mutations linked to progeria.

2. Small Molecule Medicines: Research on progeria small molecule medicines is still ongoing. These treatments may help control symptoms and enhance the lives of those who are affected.

3. Clinical Trials: To evaluate possible progeria treatments and therapies, the Progeria Research Foundation actively develops and supports clinical trials, providing encouraging paths for future treatment modalities.

Lesch-Nyhan Syndrome:

1. Allopurinol Therapy: Allopurinol treatment has been proven to be beneficial in treating hyperuricemia and uric acid overproduction, two symptoms of Lesch-Nyhan syndrome.

2. Symptomatic and Supportive Treatment: The mainstays of current Lesch-Nyhan syndrome management are symptomatic and supportive treatment, which includes individualized care plans to address the condition's particular clinical symptoms and difficulties.

To summarize, new approaches to treating Lesch-Nyhan syndrome and progeria include gene therapy, small chemical therapies, and clinical trials. These approaches may provide better ways to control and treat these uncommon genetic illnesses. Although these methods are currently in the early stages of development, they have the potential to improve the outcomes and treatment of those who are impacted by these disorders.

5.2 Promising Research Initiatives

Promising potential for the development of medicines has been demonstrated by recent research initiatives and the development of therapeutic techniques for uncommon genetic illnesses, such as Lesch-Nyhan syndrome and progeria. Among the major therapeutic approaches and research projects are:

1. Accelerated Drug Development: There are currently chances to hasten the creation of medications to cure uncommon illnesses. Globally, research centers and disease foundations are concentrating on improving knowledge of uncommon illnesses, particularly for early preclinical research.

2. Gene Therapy and Small Molecule Medicines: The possibility of gene therapy and small molecule medicines for uncommon

genetic illnesses like progeria is being investigated through ongoing research. These therapies seek to directly correct harmful mutations and control symptoms, providing possible paths toward better care and therapy.

3. Clinical studies and biomarkers: Scientists are developing novel methods for conducting clinical studies for uncommon genetic illnesses. Various strategies include the creation of safe and efficient new treatments for various illnesses, multi-center and adaptive trials, and the utilization of real-world data from wearables.

4. Individualized treatment approaches: Research groups are working to develop individualized approaches to therapy in order to address uncommon genetic illnesses such as Lesch-Nyhan syndrome and progeria. This includes making an attempt to treat the unique clinical and genetic traits of these disorders.

In conclusion, targeted therapies, individualized therapeutic approaches, and the acceleration of drug development through creative research projects and clinical trials are all possible outcomes of genetic therapies for rare genetic disorders, such as progeria and Lesch-Nyhan syndrome. The unmet medical requirements of those afflicted by these uncommon and difficult illnesses are the focus of these initiatives.

5.3 Collaborative Efforts and Global Awareness

In the realm of rare genetic illnesses, cooperative efforts and global awareness have significantly increased in the last few years. Raising awareness, promoting worldwide collaboration, and uniting the community affected by rare diseases have all been made possible by a number of organizations and projects. Important initiatives and developments in this field include the following:

1. World Rare Disease and Gene Day: Since 2009, Global Genes, a well-known

organization, has been leading the charge to empower and unite the community affected by rare diseases. With programs like Rare Disease Day, which is celebrated globally to increase awareness about rare diseases, the organization has played a key role in sustaining the momentum of worldwide awareness.

2. Research Consortium on Rare Diseases (IRDiRC): In order to meet the challenges faced by rare illnesses, the IRDiRC is a collaborative global network that seeks to locate, evaluate, support, and connect centers of expertise worldwide. This project offers a forum for research networks and organizations that focus on rare diseases to identify shared objectives and coordinate their efforts.

3. Research Collaboration and Patient Advocacy: There has been a discernible movement toward cooperative approaches that combine knowledge and resources, such as shared knowledge platforms, team science, research networks, and innovative funding structures. Crucially, patients are becoming more involved in research as sponsors and

collaborators, supporting open science, transparency, and the dismantling of geographical boundaries and data silos.

4. European Union Research and Innovation: Through a number of programs, such as collaborations with research infrastructures and the International Rare Diseases Research Consortium (IRDiRC), the European Union has been aggressively tackling rare diseases. These initiatives have improved the identification of the genes that cause rare diseases, sped up diagnosis, and improved knowledge of their natural history.

In conclusion, organizations, research consortia, and international initiatives have played a critical role in uniting the rare disease community, fostering research collaboration, and advocating for improved diagnosis and treatment of rare genetic disorders. As a result, collaborative efforts and global awareness in the field of rare genetic disorders have seen significant progress.

Conclusion

Significant progress has been made in the diagnosis, treatment, and research of uncommon genetic illnesses. The diagnosis of rare genetic illnesses in children is increasingly being done through genomic testing, and the evidence supporting long-term adoption is mounting.

Examining uncommon genetic disorders has been demonstrated to be a means of examining the role of evolutionarily conserved genes, providing a broad field for uncovering basic mechanisms necessary for human development. NGS diagnostic techniques are quickly rising to the top of the genetic diagnostic toolkit and have greatly improved the detection of uncommon diseases.

Accelerating the discovery of drugs to treat rare diseases is possible, provided that the gap between basic research and clinical interventions is addressed and there is a greater understanding of unusual disorders. Furthermore, initiatives have been undertaken to enhance the diagnosis of uncommon and undetected illnesses, emphasizing the expeditiousness of diagnosis and the scalability of genomic analysis for clinical application.

Finally, the field of uncommon genetic illnesses has greatly advanced in terms of diagnosis, treatment development, and comprehension of the basic mechanisms underlying these conditions as a result of continuous study and cooperative efforts. For those with uncommon genetic illnesses, these developments provide hope for better outcomes and treatments.

- **Recapitulation of Key Insights**

A vast spectrum of illnesses with different clinical presentations and genetic etiologies are categorized as rare genetic disorders. Important discoveries from the investigation of these illnesses include:

1. grasp the condition: In order for families to offer the right kind of support and care, they must have a complete grasp of the disease, its symptoms, and its effects on the individual's life.

2. Genetic testing: There is accumulating evidence to support the sustainable introduction of genomic testing as a standard procedure for detecting uncommon genetic illnesses in children.

3. Diagnostic advances: Almost 7,000 uncommon illnesses have been diagnosed, and many of these have a known cause. Improved characterizations of rare diseases, especially monogenic ones, have been made possible by developments in pharmacogenomics and rare illness diagnostics.

4. Drug discovery and development: Basic science and clinical treatments for uncommon genetic illnesses are significantly different from one another. The goal of ongoing research projects is to expedite the discovery of drugs to treat these ailments.

5. Collaborative efforts: scientific consortia, patient advocacy groups, and international partnerships are essential for bringing the rare

illness community together, encouraging scientific collaboration, and promoting better diagnosis and treatment of rare genetic disorders.

6. Promising research initiatives: Through creative research projects and clinical trials, the field of genetic therapeutics for uncommon genetic illnesses has hope for the creation of tailored therapeutic methods, targeted treatments, and accelerated drug development.

- **Hope and Progress in Rare Genetic Disorder Research**

Recent years have witnessed tremendous advancements in the research of uncommon genetic illnesses, providing promise for better diagnosis, treatment, and prognosis for those who are affected. Key findings from current studies include the following:

1. Better diagnoses: Developments in pharmacogenomics and rare disease diagnostics have made it possible to characterize certain illnesses—especially

monogenic ones—better. The diagnosis of rare genetic illnesses in children is increasingly being done through genomic testing, and the evidence supporting long-term adoption is mounting.

2. Drug discovery and development: There are currently chances to quicken the process of creating medications to cure uncommon illnesses. Globally, research centers and disease foundations concentrate on comprehending uncommon ailments better, and current research projects seek to expedite the creation of drugs to treat these conditions.

3. Collaborative efforts: Research consortia, patient advocacy groups, and international collaborations are essential for bringing the rare illness community together, encouraging research collaboration, and promoting better diagnosis and treatment of rare genetic disorders.

4. Promising research initiatives: Through creative research projects and clinical trials, the field of genetic therapeutics for uncommon

genetic illnesses has hope for the creation of tailored therapeutic methods, targeted treatments, and accelerated drug development.

In conclusion, there is hope for better outcomes and therapies for those impacted by rare genetic disorders, thanks to the continued research and cooperative efforts in this area. Research on rare genetic disorders has a bright future thanks to developments in diagnosis, medication development, and discovery, as well as cooperative efforts and exciting new projects.

Reference

An overview of rare genetic disorders and recent diagnostic. Saudi Journal for Health Sciences.

Clinical Features of the Lesch-Nyhan Syndrome. JAMA Internal Medicine.

Lesch Nyhan Syndrome - Symptoms, Causes, Treatment. NORD.

Topics by Science.gov: Lesch-Nyhan Syndrome. Science.gov.

International Lesch-Nyhan Disease Association. National Organization for Rare Disorders.

About Author

Dr. Gerrard Andrews is a multifaceted professional with a diverse background in research and writing. His career has encompassed several areas of expertise, including literature, genetics, and hydrology. As an author and researcher, Dr. Andrews has made significant contributions to the understanding of African American literature, 18th- and 19th-century African American writing, and the African American slave narrative tradition. In the field of genetics, he has been a prominent figure in molecular biology and gerontology, with a focus on searching for a cure for aging and identifying genes related to human aging. Additionally, Dr. Andrews has also been involved in teaching and supervisory roles, demonstrating his commitment to education and leadership in various scientific domains. His wide-ranging work reflects a deep and enduring dedication to scholarship and research in multiple disciplines.